Disclaimer for New Weight Loss and Prevent Diabetes Guide for 2017!

The Proven Weight Loss and Prevent Diabetes Tips. No Slimming Pills and Side Effects. If we are healthy, the world belongs to us.

All the information presented in the following eBook: The New Weight Loss and Prevent Diabetes Guide For 2017 and links from this book are for **educational** and **resource** purposes only.

The information in this text is to help you make informed decisions about weight loss and diabetes prevention. It is NOT a substitute for or an addition to any advice given to you by your physician or qualified health care professional.

I'm 44 years old now and I suffered from severe constipation for many years. After taking doctor medicine does not solve my constipation problems. I ever hospitalized before from severe constipation. Thanks to 65FruitieFibre® Probiotics supplement. As for now, I no longer have constipation and fully recovered from severe constipation. I then introduced this product to my friend who is 66 years old. He suffered from severe constipation too for more than 40 years. After taking 65FruitieFibre® Probiotics for less than a month, his constipation problem resolved. My friend and I are indeed very grateful and thankful for this amazing product.

Ms Grace Lee, 5 Jan 2017

Before having 65FruitieFibre® Probiotics, I always felt bloated, not much appetite and had trouble going to toilet. I tried different type / brand of detox supplements before but the results won't last after 1 box. Chance upon 65FruitieFibre® Probiotics and decided to give it a try. It reduced my bloatedness, surprisingly increased my appetite and it definitely ease my constipation (from 3 - 4 days to 3 - 4 times per day). Even though I didn't lose any weight, I did maintain my current weight while having more meals and late night supper. It is definitely affordable and effective as compared to those on shelf products which cost much more and less effective.

Ms Cecelia Seah, 3 Jan 2017

So far 65FruitieFibre® Probiotics is going well for me. It does clear out my skin breakout issue. I stopped having massive breakouts and of course I no longer have constipation. I'm glad I came across this product. I used to pile up foundation to cover things up on my face, now I don't put anything on my face and my skin actually looks normal. I used to buy many facial products to fix the breakout problem and none of them worked until I came across 65FruitieFibre® Probiotics. Very impressed. Will definitely repurchase. Thank you so much for the excellent service!

Ms Nora Faiqa, 18 Dec 2016

I got to know this product through word of mouth with good reviews. Hence, I decided to give it a try as I have mild constipation issue. Aft subsequent intake of the drink before I sleep, it really helps to regulate my bowel movement (sometimes twice a day) and my stomach will feel less bloated. I'm quite impressed!

Ms Amanda Kuan

Going to toilet more for the first time, then back to usual, also can spot some black stuffs with the waste, will continue to consume as I believe it will help my health. It is a great product that is why I continue to consume it.

Ms Cindy Tiew

Initially I have no idea about this 65FruitieFibre product, but one of my Chinese friend who suffered certain cancer in China, and her Doctor suggest her to take this as supplementary, she followed the suggestion and consumed several boxes already. Will continue to consume it. Highly recommended.

Ms Yuan

My tummy do become smaller a bit and i do lose bit of weight too. Will continue consume it till reach my ideal weight.

Mr Kosey Low

YOUR
HEALTHY
CHOICE
65果汁纤维

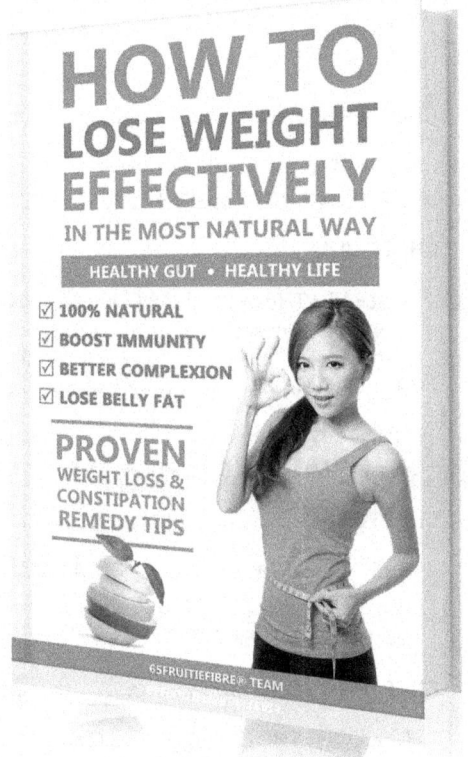

WWW.65FRUITIEFIBRE.SG

TABLE OF CONTENTS

Had it with strict diets? Ever thought of losing weight naturally? **WITH EVERLASTING RESULTS?**

YES, YOU ARE ON THE RIGHT PLACE!

If you are one of those who keeps up with contemporary studies in food and nutrition, you must have heard about probiotics and prebiotics. You might know that they **assist digestion** and turn down **bloating**, as urged in numerous **yogurt commercials** on TV. But you might not know any other benefits of these.

It must be shocking for you to perceive that probiotics are real: **"BACTERIA"** whereas **prebiotic** is the food that **probiotics** live on. Although after realizing it some of you might feel disgusted, but learning it is the first step for the **apprehension** of how hospitable these bacteria are for us. If the idea of bacteria in the gut still makes you jiggle, hold your breath to know that some of these bacteria are our friends. The childhood knowledge of bacteria making us ill might make it difficult for you to digest that there are actually some **GOOD bacteria** which hold immense importance in our health.

The World Health Organization (WHO) defines probiotics as **"living organisms which, when administered in adequate amounts, confer a health benefit on the host."**

Diabetic patients often have weak immune system, because of high glucose level in blood. Adding **Probi-**

otics to the diet helps boost our immune system, by communicating with immune cells to initiate a strike against harmful bacteria.

Not only does these probiotics challenge diabetes, they are helpful in many other health issues, mostly in, **Alleviating lactose intolerance, fighting irritable bowel syndrome and preventing urinary tract infections.**

Most of you are aware by now that foods that offer probiotics have a long list of health benefits, but nonetheless, prebiotic foods are still to be discovered. **SADLY,** most of us do not consume prebiotic on regular basis, which has led to destructive results including aggravated indigestion, higher levels of inflammation, lower immune function, higher likelihood of **weight gain** and a raised risk for various chronic diseases. While probiotics help in the well-being of the **gut,** prebiotics help nourish probiotics. By operating them together, you can achieve an even better result.

FOOD comprising high levels of probiotics include **YOGURT, BUTTER-CREAM** and **COTTAGE CHEESE.** While PREBIOTICS are found in under **ripe bananas, raw jicama, and acacia gum** easily found in our near about.

Yes! It's true that in our busy life we forget about our health. Don't have time to look for what to eat and what not. And still:

"Looking For an Effective Weight Loss or Slimming Solution But Worried About the Side Effects of Slimming Pills?"

If you are looking at how to lose weight fast naturally and effectively **65FruitieFibre®** Probiotics fiber is the most effective weight loss and slimming solutions for you!

It does not cause any side effects as the ingredients are all natural, contains fruits and vegetables which 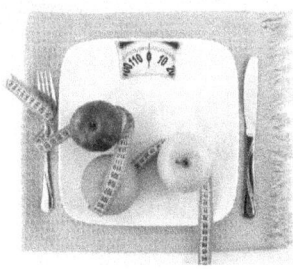 are rich in Vitamin C to promote beautiful skin complexion, no chemical, no preservative, no drug content, thus it is 100% safe for long term consumption.

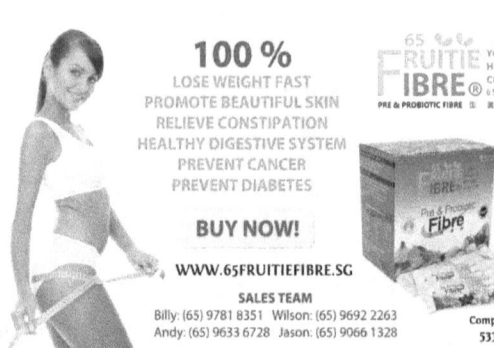
"**65fruitiefibre®** Probiotics detoxes and provides nutritional needs for our body. Fat builds up to protect from toxins that build up in our body. Removing toxins is needed to promote better overall health, to lose weight and maintain a **slim** and **beautiful body**!"

Our clients have been using 65FruitieFibre® Probiotics and that's what they have to say:

"After I regularly consume this 65FruitieFibre® Probiotics fibre

*product daily, till date I have **effectively lose my weight around 7 kg!** My blood sugar level reduced to a healthy range too. Highly Recommended! - Mr. Jason, 1 Aug 2016"*

SO HOW 65FRUITIEFIBRE® PREBIOTICS AND PROBIOTICS ARE HELPFUL TO US?

There are numerous benefits including:

- ➢ **Diabetes prevention.**
- ➢ **Weight loss.**
- ➢ **Increase energy.**
- ➢ **Stronger immune system.**
- ➢ **Improved digestion.**
- ➢ **Healthier skin, since probiotics naturally treat eczema and psoriasis.**

- ➢ Reduced cold and flu.

- ➢ Healing from leaky gut syndrome and inflammatory bowel disease.

- ➢ Preventing and treating urinary tract infections.

- ➢ Healing inflammatory bowel conditions.

- ➢ Fighting food-borne illnesses.

- ➢ Managing and preventing eczema in children.

- ➢ Battle cancer.

- ➢ Treat kidney stones.

- ➢ Prevent cavities and gum disease.

- ➢ Treat colitis and Crohn's disease.

- ➢ Combat antibiotic resistant bacteria.

- ➢ Treat liver disease.

- ➢ Lower cholesterol.

- ➢ Manage autism.

- ➢ Fight bacteria that causes ulcers.

And more ...

Chapter 1

WHY SHOULD WE LOSE WEIGHT FAST AND EFFECTIVELY IN THE MOST NATURAL WAY?

Being overweight does not only make you look ugly but it is also detrimental to your personal health. Obese people are more likely to encounter high blood pressure and the **high cholesterol level** that can lead to heart strokes or even diabetes. Although when we talk about being obese or carrying a lot of fats, we relate it to heart diseases or diabetes. Forgetting it for a moment and thinking more about it, rigorously being overweight might cause you to suffer joint pains of-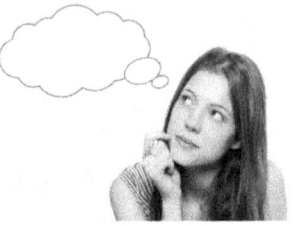ten named as **"Osteoarthritis"**. In this, the bones cartilage slowly destroys making joints unbearably painful.

One more awful epidemic lead by fats is sleep apnea, where your breath keeps on blocking again and again. Making you have uncomfortable sleep. It happens due to fats deposited in airways.

For obese women, it is difficult to have a normal **childbirth**. They might have more medical procedures and **cesarean Chapter**. Lastly being fat. Makes one more vulnerable to **cancer.**

Sleep Apnea - The millions of people suffering from respiratory problems and sleep associated with sleep apnea. Like other diseases and risk factors mentioned above, you can stop breathing during sleep, preventing and combating when you reach and maintain a healthy weight.

Everyone knows that the risk factors for the life-threatening encounter with excess weight. Risk factors increase with weight gain. If these risk factors do not scare you should.

Take as much as possible to prevent and stop the work.

Ask yourself again, why should you lose weight? I hope this article has helped answer that question.

If you could lose 10 or 50 pounds, and now is the time to love your body, love your life. Take time to love yourself and be amazed at how much better you will feel and how much better your relationships can be?

To Be Happier - weight loss, when done in a responsible way, and certainly benefit the physical, emotional and spiritual health as well. One of the first things a dieter report is the amount of excess energy you have after losing up to 5 or 10

million pounds. They also sleep better and enjoy better sex lives.

Author's Recommendation

To obtain a healthy lifestyle, we highly recommend 65FruitieFibre® Probiotics to include in your daily diet to help weight loss and prevent constipation effectively which lead to colon cancer, visit www.65FruitieFibre.sg

Chapter 2

UNLEASH THE SECRET OF HIGHLY RECOMMENDED CONSTIPATION REMEDY TIPS

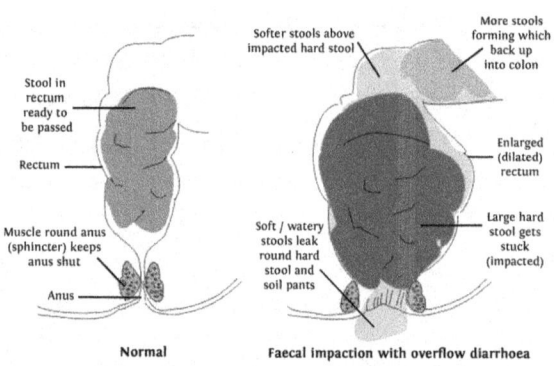

Normal   Faecal impaction with overflow diarrhoea

Constipation is a medical condition-in which a person is unable to pass the bowel for at least a week or passes a small amount of bowel less than three times. Many people affected with this condition experience some frustrating and even embarrassing moments that affect their daily lives.

However, many of them do not know if they are already experiencing constipation and this is an alarming truth. They would only realize that they are already experiencing constipation when they have felt the worst of their signs. Therefore, curing this condition would already involve medical help, when in fact, they could have relieved by just changing their diet. In **infants**, constipation can be a very distressing experience and this involves careful evaluation of parents. The natural cause of constipation is the mainly **poor diet** that is aggravated by poor or too little exercise and fecal stasis in the **colon**.

Common symptoms experienced by people suffering from constipation include discomfort and pain in the passage of hardened stools, firm and distended **abdomen**, and the need to defecate becomes less.

Often, a change in diet facilitates constipation. However, there are conditions in which people who experience constipation need medical help to relieve constipation. A **laxative** is a common drug that is given to a person who has constipation, either by mouth or by suppository.

Causes of Constipation:

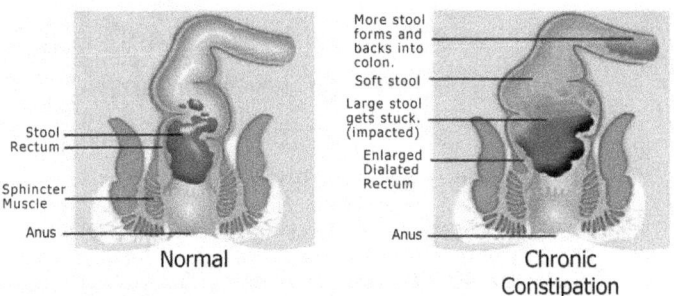

Normal

Chronic
Constipation

Poor nutrition and sedentary life-style with lack of exercise are the two causes of constipation discussed above. Those who like to eat foods low in fiber are at greater risk of being constipated. Foods rich in fiber can be found in whole **grains**, **vegetables** and **fruits** like papaya, mango and oranges. These varieties of foods are recommended to people who love to eat **high-fat foods**.

Although babies are not constipated, the transition from **breastfeeding** to bottle feeding or formula can cause the baby to develop constipation. Since the addition of fiber-rich foods to babies' diets is not a good way to relieve constipation, parents are expected to monitor the process of eliminating their babies. Constipation relief measures vary between age groups, therefore, there is a need for individualized care or management.

Another cause of constipation is the **lack of water** intake. Drinking water not only means drinking eight glasses of water each day also means adding juices to our daily drink. However, we must be **cautious** about what type of liquids we are taking, because there are also those that can cause constipation, such as milk drinks and soft drinks. In infants, the most common cause of constipation is a formula-fed diet with a low or poor fluid intake. Adding more liquid to a **baby's diet** can help resolve constipation. Also, babies or even adults who abuse various medications, including laxatives or **purgatives**, may soon develop constipation and later become dependent on these medications. Parents are instructed to seek medical help when their child is experiencing difficulty passing stools for a week as this may involve more complicated conditions and appropriate measures to be taken.

There are also medical conditions that can lead to constipation. And a condition called irritable bowel syn drome, which produces soft stools and a few natural episodes, or recurrent abdominal pain can lead to constipation. This is usually found turbulence in children from **6 months to 3 years**. Other colon problems can also lead to constipation, such as a disease or lack of ten years **hirschsprung megacolon**. Adults who suffer from inertia or afflicted with back injuries and strokes may encounter constipation. Also diseases like lupus, diabetes, a disease that can lead to intestinal disease.

When food is slowed down through the intestine or stopped, constipation develops. **Medical Research** said that more water is absorbed from the food we eat because it

puts in the large intestine. The result is a stool drier and more difficult to eject. Slow down the process
of digestion, and is said to be
caused by certain diseases, and take
medications and changes in diet.

Natural Cures Constipation:

It is easy to understand the importance of treating natural constipation. Therefore, it is necessary to
read to know the different options
for you.

1. Make the change in your diet

Switching to your diet is one that is
rich in fruits and vegetables like carrots, peas, sweet potatoes, leafy
greens, peaches, oranges perhaps
one of the best natural constipation
remedies you can do to get rid of

constipation. By doing so, you provide the body with an adequate amount of fiber, bran and thus it is much easier to defecate.

2. Take probiotics supplements

Probiotics are one of the most effective supplements in helping to relieve constipation and get rid of constipation.

"Can probiotics really relieve constipation? "

The intestines are comprised of billions and billions of bacteria, so when a disproportion occurs during these levels of bacteria (known as dysbiosis) it leads to digestive symptoms, such as constipation. The majority of bacteria that makes up our large intestine are the Bifidobacteria and Lactobacillus species, therefore it is practical that probiotics with specific strains owed to these species are generally regarded as most beneficial in assisting constipation. Some probiotics produce lactic acid and short-chain fatty acids (SCFAs) that lower the ph level in the colon which heightens muscle contractions along the colon (peristalsis) to enhance regularity.

Some Bifidobacterium and Lactobacillus species can enhance bowel regularity and mucous secretion by changing bound bile salts into free bile salts. These types of free bile salts cause more water to be pulled into the bowel which softens the stools and aids in constipation.

3. Drink water

Water is the best and most effective of all natural constipation remedies there. Water provides a lot of benefits, one of which is keeping the stool soft and moist. In addition, water can keep the body hydrated. Making the body work better.

Some other tips:

Flaxseed is rich in fiber and a lack of fiber is one of the main reasons that people suffer from constipation.

Psyllium husk and we are surprised that this is not mentioned often in different lists for physical therapy constipation, but it is a great gift to treat constipation. It also helps to put pressure on the **colon walls**, muscles and contracted stool can easily pass through.

Olive oil is a great constipation soldier as it has the function of a natural laxative and filled with many of the essential **fatty acids**.

Cascara sagrada is a helpful treatment that provides relief from constipation. It is also non-addictive and nutritionally beneficial to the stomach, liver, pancreas and gallbladder. It works as a natural colon cleanser, and thus keeps the body's protection from toxic losses and fecal matter.

Bael fruit is an excellent choice for the treatment of constipation. And it is considered the best laxative among all other fruits. It really is a wonderful constipation delight. It has the ability to cleanse the digestive tract along with great relief from constipation. It is also useful to put the natural as well as chronic constipation problems.

Guava can be eaten to get relief from the problem of constipation. It is necessary to eat foods with guava seeds to combat the problem of constipation. In addition, it is possible to have orange, papaya, peaches, pears and grapes to promote the health of the digestive system.

Bran cereal can be used as an effective constipation treatment and is ideal for young children and adolescents. To treat the problem of constipation, you can use **corn syrup** mixed with water. This traditional treatment to relieve constipation includes honey or sugar in a full glass of milk. Drinking twice in a day can certainly make you free from the problem problem of constipation.

You can choose from a lot of constipation remedies there, but natural is always better. Nor should we forget that other diseases can be observed by constipation. Therefore, it is still better to consult a doctor to make sure there is no serious condition that is causing your constipation.

"Do you know, colon cleansing procedures cost can be as high as $1400? Prevention is always better than cure. Probiotics supplement aid constipation and prevent colon cancer"

Claim your full bundle eBook (PDF, AZW and Kindle version) at:
http://ebook.65fruitiefibre.sg/bundle

Chapter 3

UNLEASH THE SECRET OF HIGHLY RECOMMENDED WEIGHT LOSS TIPS

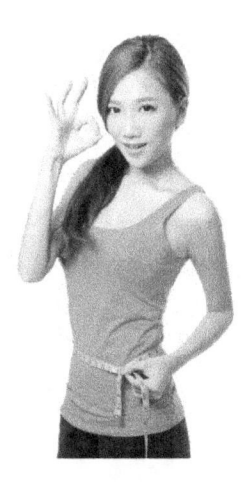

Yes, it's always easy to start with a diet plan, but it's always difficult to keep up with it. For that, you must be motivated and have goals in your mind. Goals which will finally take you to success. You will never be advised to lose weight, by eating nothing or go on a fad diet.

The best way to start is to know yourself first. To know what are your eating habits and what are the loopholes in your diet leading to obesity.

Try not to be sluggish, keep your body in movement. Be active.

Control your urge of hunger. Say No to the high- calorie foods provided and choose the lowest calorie con-taining diet.

Drink 8 glass of water a day. This will increase your metabolic rate and also feels your full belly. So will eat less.

Beverage calories liberation. Cutting soda or sweetened iced tea and any drink is full of calories. They do little to satisfy hunger and add tons of calories that are not necessary.

Cut refined carbohydrates for a period of two weeks. Your body can become dependent on food items such as white bread, baked goods, refined foods and this can make the body fat burner ineffective.

Take carbohydrates in AM and protein at the PM. Change from simple carbohydrates is one more effective of the weight loss tips that can happen to you to lose weight quickly. Over the next two weeks, keeping the carbohydrates from your diet after lunch and not only release a lot of excess weight of water, but also the body forced to burn more fat in the body to get energy fast as the source (i.e. carbohydrates) are not available.

Avoid snacks at night or have protein or vegetables. To maximize your weight loss you want to avoid snacks late at night, but if you're really hungry physically have or plant protein, these foods do not renewed insulin that can prevent fat burning overnight level.

Are you used to of eating when boredom strikes? Then you must control that. That's the worst we can do to our self. Instead of eating in your free time make sure to do something productive, go for a walk or do some chores around the house.

Lastly be honest to yourself and be promising. If you've left the track, go back to it.

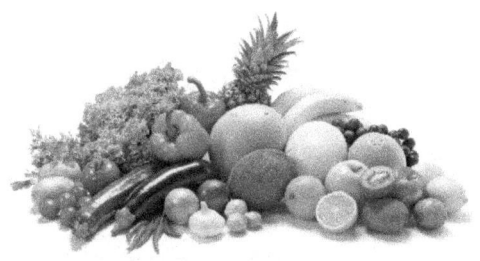

Let's come to the most difficult part of our diet plan!

How to eat less when the heart wants more?

i. Eat slowly and take smaller bites.

ii. Eat many times a day but don't take in high calorie and fat food. Food consumption after every 2 hours is recommended

iii. Eat healthy food like fruits vegetables whole grains fish or even dried peas.

iv. Make sure to use oil lesser in your diet and try making food with baking and boiling.

v. Before accepting any food count its calorie and sugar count and avoid high calorie and sugar products.

vi.   Avoid bakery products.

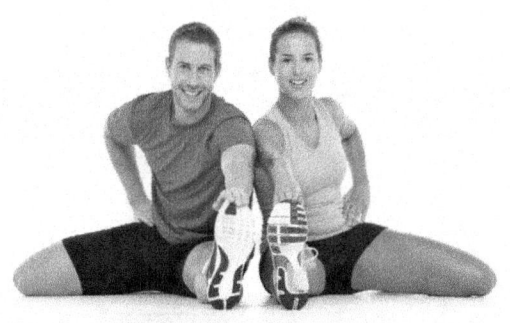

Apart from **diet plans** exercise is also worthwhile for the body. Make sure you are giving your body the right time and right type of exercise.

Regular exercise can keep you safe from a heart attack, stroke, high blood pressure and other health problems. An exercise of **150 minutes** is most favorable for an adult or minimum of **75 minutes**. Exercise will help you combat deadly diseases and increase your **metabolic rate** making you lose weight quickly and effectively.

Author's Recommendation

To obtain a healthy lifestyle, we highly recommend 65FruitieFibre® Probiotics to include in your daily diet to help weight loss and prevent constipation effectively which lead to colon cancer, visit www.65FruitieFibre.sg

Chapter 4

UNLEASH THE SECRET OF CONTROLLING DIABETES WITH PRE AND PROBIOTICS

Day after day new studies is advancing in this century. And same is the case when a research proved that pre and probiotics can help prevent diabetes. Especially if one is dealing with type 2 diabetes and **pre-diabetes** which are considered by insulin resistance or glucose intolerance.

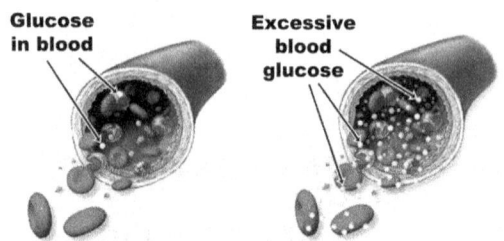

We talk about insulin resistance when the insulin receptors on cell halt to accepting hormone insulin, due to which cells stop accepting the intake of glucose in them making them selfless energetic which causes a person to feel fatigued and blood glucose level raised.

Glucose intolerance in referred to when body cells become intolerant to glucose itself and don't allow glucose to pass through cell membrane. Blood sugar is normalized in diabetic patients when probiotics are used regularly.

Probiotics include strains of lactobacillus, further preference lactobacillus acidophilus, and L.rhamno-
sus.

If You Are Looking For Buying Probiotics Supplements, Make Sure These Things Are In Your Mind!

1. Make sure while choosing a probiotic that it contains at least a 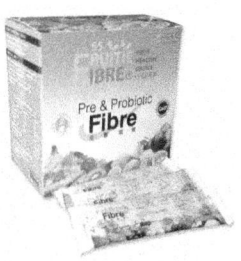 strain of L. acidophilus, L. Fermentum, L.rhamnosus, B. longum, and B. bifidum. Although yeast is good for gut health, but when choosing

supplements avoid having yeast in it. Choose a supplement which is enteric coated so that stomach acid cannot destroy useful bacteria in it.

2.   The most obvious step is to check the expiration date.

3.   Check the quality of your prebiotics.

4.   Make sure it contain at least a least of 25 billion Colony Forming Units (CFU's).

5.   Lastly, talk to your pharmacist before you start taking the probiotics supplements.

Claim your full bundle eBook (PDF, AZW and Kindle version) at:
http://ebook.65fruitiefibre.sg/bundle

Chapter 5

UNLEASH THE SECRET OF HIGHLY RECOMMENDED DIABETIC CONTROL TIPS

"Diabetes is a marathon, Not a Sprint".

Probiotics are essential for everyone, **young and old**. Studies have proven that regular consumption of Probiotics helps to control and **prevent diabetes**. Before starting any race you must know what the starting point is. So people. Here, before you start applying diabetic control tips on yourself, see where you stand right now. Know about your weight, calorie count and glucose count in the blood.

Here comes the 2nd step, after you know where you stand, start keeping a record of your daily activity. That will make you realize how much you have exerted today. After this, start applying our recommended tips on you. Make sure you bring your own **homemade lunch** to the work, which is included with healthy **nutrients** as advised later in the book.

Let's change the daily routine now. Instead of choosing a highly creamed latte on a café try choosing a **coffee** made of **low-fat milk**.

So what to do when we are at our favorite restaurant. Try choosing **grilled food** with salad.

Keep this sincere advice to yourself if you are thinking to combat diabetes. Always, keep a pedometer fastened with your clothes, so you can keep a control on the daily number of steps taken by you. A person must take **10,000 steps** a day for a sound body.

Do you feel hungry when it's not even the meal time? Obviously, you'll grab a bunch of crisps or any junk food. Let's replace it with a "**Sugar-Free Bubblegum**". Do you often go to a market and choose a typical sort of veggie or fruit? From now on, try the different type of vegetable and fruit every week.

A full plate of the meal makes you feel happy, isn't? But if it's a big full plate that is really bad for your health. Replace the big plate with a smaller one. The full small plate will still make it soothing to your eyes with less meal eaten by you.

Last and not the least in actual, keep a check on your **blood sugar** every two hours.

Tips for the Care of Patients with Diabetes

1. Keep control of blood glucose in the blood regularly as suggested by your doctor.

2. You must take prescribed medication or insulin dose regularly.

3. Regular exercise is useful in controlling glucose levels. However, you should avoid these exercises that can cause additional complications such as cardiovascular disease, hypoglycemia, etc.

4. You must lose some extra weight because weight loss dramatically helps control diabetes.

5. Stop alcohol and quitting smoking.

6. You should avoid foods that contain sugar and follow your meal plan for diabetes.

7. You should avoid stress, fear, and anger.

These are not myths, studies have proven probiotics help to control and prevent diabetes.

Author's Recommendation

To obtain a healthy lifestyle, we highly recommend 65FruitieFibre® Probiotics to include in your daily diet to help weight loss and prevent constipation effectively which lead to colon cancer, visit www.65FruitieFibre.sg

THE POWER OF PROBIOTICS THAT MAKE YOU ACHIEVE EVERLASTING WEIGHT LOSS AND DIABETIC PREVENTION

In this century, obesity inflamed liver and type 2 diabetes are becoming a tremendous epidemic. Recent researchers have now shown that pro and prebiotics can actually make one fight these plagues with no side effects.

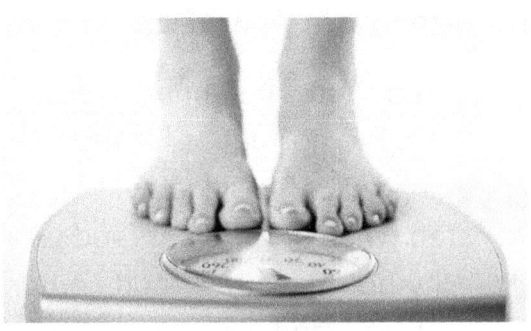

But how?

Bacteria, as our concept of bad bacteria, is changed now, there are also good bacteria living in our body. These good bacteria live in our colon named as "Bifido-bacteria". These bacteria aid weight loss when probiotics are ingested.

But the bad bacteria helps increase body fat when fatty food is taken. So it's always recommended choosing food with more probiotics which will eventually make good bacteria help to lose your weight.

When you are hungry and take food, the hormones hit the signal of being full. This signal will be generated when any type of food is taken. Why not make this food comprising prebiotic and probiotic fiber. As it will certainly control the craving.

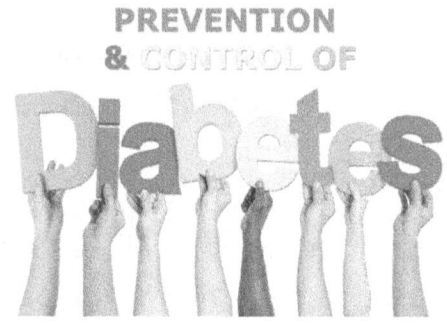

Claim your full bundle eBook (PDF, AZW and Kindle version) at:
http://ebook.65fruitiefibre.sg/bundle

Chapter 7

DISCOVER THE CASE STUDIES ON CONSTIPATION REMEDY WITH PRE AND PROBIOTICS

In our previous part, we discussed on constipation, its causes and remedies that are helpful in

MOST NATURAL WAY OF CONSTIPATION REMEDY ? "PRE AND PROBIOTICS"

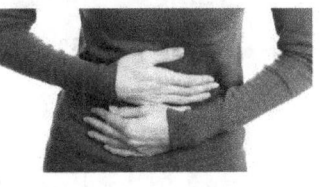

constipation cure. But, what about Prebiotics and Probiotics? Does Prebiotics and Prebiotics help in curing consti-pation?

Yes, taking probiotics for constipation boosts **bowel movement**. Probiotics are micro-organisms or friendly bacteria that help to keep the digestive tract healthy among other health benefits. However, it is important to note that different probiotic products contain different strains of bacteria, which perform different functions. That is why you should pick your probiotics supplements or products carefully.

Studies show that Lactobacillus **paracasei** strain is very helpful in treating constipation and restoring normal bowel movement. So you should look for a product that contains this particular strain. You should also read the label very well to ensure that it stipulates that the bacteria strains are 'live'.

Although taking probiotics for constipation works, it is also important to add that probiotics cannot survive for long in your gut without the right food to feed on. Remember that these are living organisms and all living organisms need food for sustenance. That is where prebiotics come in.

Prebiotics are dietary fibers that serve as food for the good bacteria; they also help to clean up the digestive tract to make it conducive for the probiotics to work effectively.

Moreover, prebiotics are also proven to help to enhance digestion, reduce bloating, and boost the immune system among many other benefits. In other words, taking probiotics for constipation works better if taken with a high-quality prebi-otics.

Case Studies about Prebiotic and Probiotic to Prevent Colon Cancer

Previous studies have indicated that the general population of 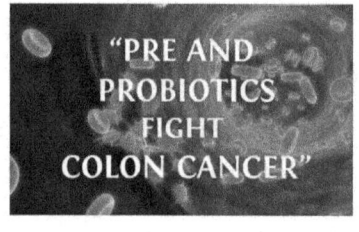 intestinal bacteria associated with the onset of colon cancer through the production of carcinogens and companions of **carcinogens**, or **pro-carcinogens**. An earlier study reported that only 20% of the animals are germ-free and offered to devel-op chemically induced colon tu-mors, compared to 93% of their counterparts with normal flora.

Abnormal use caused by foci of azoxymethane crypts in mice, Reddy et al. I have found that stimulating the growth of bifidobacteria in the colon can lead to inhibition of colon carcinogenesis. The authors suggested that the inhibition of aberrant crypt foci and crypt multiplicity is attributed to the effect of lowering the pH of the bifidobacteria in the colon, which hinders the subsequent growth of E. coli and Clostridium.

It may be lower in the growth of these pathogenic microorganisms of the disease also occurs the formation of bacterial enzymes such as beta-glucuronidase, which can convert procarcinogens to the proximal carcinogens.

ANTI CANCER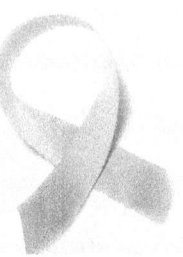

These **anticancer** properties also studied at the molecular level.

There are fifty-seven cytochrome P450 encoded in the human genome, primarily stimulating the metabolism of steroids, bile acids, Aakozanoad, drugs and extraterrestrial biology chemicals. However, some of the P450s are also carcinogenic active.

Recent epidemiological research has shown an increased risk of colon cancer in individuals with high P4501A2 activity.

I assume that the **metabolism** of heterocyclic amines activate carcinogens transmitted by colon food in humans is produced by oxidation followed by O-N-acetylation to form N-acetoxy arylamine which binds to DNA to give carcinogenic **DNA adducts**.

And these hepatic cytochrome P4501A2 and acetyl-2 (NAT-2) steps were stimulated, respectively. It was found that probiotics such misery can reduce the risk of colon cancer, through the production of metabolites that can affect the mixed function of P450s and later affect to convert azoxymethane from the proximal end to the carcinogen in the end. This led to the suggestion that **microorganisms** can suppress colon cancer.

In-depth research also showed that **cultured milk** has desmutagenicity. This increased activity with a viable cell number increased, indicating that probiotic work plays an important role in inhibition of mutations.

Thyagaraja and Hosono found that the microorganisms isolated from the "**spectator**", the traditional grain pulse of India can exert desmutagenicity on various mutagenic products, heterocyclic amines and mycotoxins.

Further studies on the desmutagenicity of probiotic properties indicate that the **desmutagenic** materials may be present in the cell envelope of the bacterial cell wall.

It was found on the wall of B-cell clay to inhibit tumor activity in a mouse peritoneal cells in the vitro preparation, while they were found in the cell wall of the dead heat preparation L. casei (LC9018) to induce Immunity against tumor induction in the randomized and controlled comparative study of 223 phase III and cervical cancer patients. Antitumor effects were found due to the activation of macrophages by LC9018.

In addition, it was suggested that they may bind to the cell wall of probiotics. This has been supported by previous studies that found bound by the skeletal parts of the cell wall of probiotics at the junction of the mutagen and heterocyclic amines that probiotic intestinal properties. In addition, it has also been found in whole bifidobacteria cells to connect with carcinogenic 3-amino-1,4-dimethyl-5 H-pyrido [4,3-b] indole carcinogen, and thus physically removed by carcinogenic methylazoxymethanol.

Feces and then reducing their absorption in the intestinal cavity.

Other studies have assumed that probiotics have protective effects against **colon cancer** by changing the process of differentiation of cancer cells. The use of a colonized human colon cancer cell line (HT-29), Baricault et al. To study the effect of **fermented milk** on the growth of colon cancer cells. Fermented milk with individual strains of Lactobacillus helveticus, misery, L. acidophilus or a combination of contractual freedom and L. delbrueckii subsp. Bulgari. Aggregated

HT-29 cells later in fermented milk, researchers found that 10-50% of HT-29 cells showed a decrease in growth. The analysis also revealed that specific activities of a specific marker of HT-29 cell differentiation, such as dipeptidyl peptides increased. The authors suggested that cancer cells have entered the process of differentiation leading to less growth.

Author's Recommendation

To obtain a healthy lifestyle, we highly recommend 65FruitieFibre® Probiotics to include in your daily diet to help weight loss and prevent constipation effectively which lead to colon cancer, visit www.65FruitieFibre.sg

Chapter 8

DISCOVER THE CASE STUDIES ON HOW PRE AND PROBIOTICS HELP TO PREVENT DIABETES

So is it really possible that consuming pre and probiotics will help cut sugar level in a body? Following researches would help you to seek the answer.

RESEARCH 1

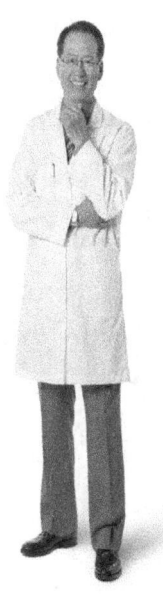

A research carried out in **Griffith University Australia** and central **Queensland University** conducted a quantitative analysis test for the effects of probiotics on blood glucose level. 14 clinical studies were carried out to test the blood glucose level of people who were treated with pre and probiotics.

The research was carried out in various ways,

some were done with only one particular species of probiotics, some
with one type of prebiotics and others were carried out with both of
them together. These research took
a lot of time with some ending **six
weeks** and others **28 weeks**.

All tests were carried in the morning
before breakfast. And the meta-
analysis concluded that the results
were consistent in every way.

RESEARCH 2

Research in Cornell University carried out by **Prof. John March**. They
researched on a strain of probiotics
"**lactobacillus bacteria**" found in the
human gut, for its assistance in

controlling blood sugar.

GLP-1 is a hormone that increases **insulin production**. In this research, tests were carried out to prove how lactobacillus which secretes GLP-1 activate intestinal epithelial cells into insulin secreting cells in both humans and rats. Therefore, hormones secreting **GLP-1** were given orally to rats who were suffering from diabetes for a 90 days period. And a group of control rats was given normal lactobacillus strain.

The results showed that the diabetic rats were given GLP-1 secreting **probiotics had 30 % lower** chance of high blood sugar. The upper intestinal epithelial cells started behaving like pancreatic cells by **monitoring blood** glucose level and keeps **insulin production** up to required amount needed for optimal blood **glucose level**. Interestingly no effect was observed when probiotics were given to healthy rats. Hence the result proved the whole experiment positively.

Claim your full bundle eBook (PDF, AZW and Kindle version) at:
http://ebook.65fruitiefibre.sg/bundle

DISCOVER THE CASE STUDIES ON HOW PRE AND PROBIOTICS HELPS TO LOSE WEIGHT FAST AND EFFECTIVELY

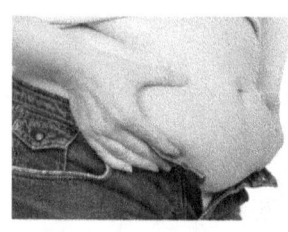 A research was carried out by Virginia Tech, in which 20 healthy men were said to take high-calorie diet and high-fat diet for four weeks. One group was given milkshake high in **probiotics** with a **strain** of **lactobacillus** while other acted as a control.

At the end of the experiment men taking probiotics were found to have lower body mass and fat gain. Thus, proved, that taking **probiotics pills** in routine diet would help regulate body fat **accumulation** making one lose weight easily. Another research gathered **around 120 people**, dealing with inches of fat around the tummy and hip were seen to cut inches of fats when provided with probiotics diet. But it was concluded that those who left taking probiotics, **regained weight after some time**.

The role of prebiotic in weight loss:

Prebiotics can be very useful when trying to lose a few calories. Prebiotic supplements for weight loss help reduce appetite and make you feel full quickly. Since weight gain and food go hand in hand and suppress the desire to eat will be vital in reducing weight.

These supplements work on certain hormones in the body, giving you a sense of satisfaction. Thus, the bacteria helps suppress appetite, and therefore, will not feel the need to eat. This leads to weight loss. Most foods that contain prebiotics also be fiber. This is the reason that probiotics are essential for optimal health. Sometimes, they can help you lose weight because you are sure to improve bowel movement, and this will keep the digestive system clean. Fiber is a volume in the diet because it helps to absorb nutrients quickly helps to suppress the desire to eat. Again, you will be able to reduce appetite and eventually you will lose weight.

Prebiotics help to increase the good bacteria and reduce harmful naturally. This helps to prevent infections. For maximum benefits, it should consume foods such as whole kiwi skin, raw oats, raw onions, raw honey and raw artichoke. For greater impact, you have to eat at least two kiwifruits a day.

The best solution is to use a kiwi supplement. Most of them come from the pulp and lyophilized to provide the minimum of the active ingredients. Various supplements are created differently. When choosing supplements prebiotic, there are some factors to consider. Annex should. I found naturally in foods, and is extracted at low temperatures to preserve the enzymes are enzymes, phenol, fiber and contain no chemical additives.

A Comparison between Antibiotic & Probiotics;

Which Is BETTER?

Definition: Probiotic vs. Antibiotic

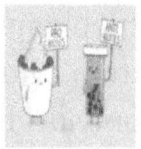

- Probiotics are defined as a group of live bacteria which are known to bring health benefits to the host. The term probiotic comes from the Latin preposition, "*pro*" (meaning for) and Greek word "*bios*" (meaning life). So, it literally means "*for life*".
- Antibiotics refer to any substance that is produced, they are a microorganism that acts against the growth of other microorganisms. This term is derived from the Greek words "*anti*" (meaning against) and "*bios*" (meaning life). Thus, it literally means "*against life*".

The antibiotics are used to prevent the growth of bacteria. There is some concern about bacterial resistance to antibiotics. What we call "super bugs" or those born of resistance to antibiotics. Probiotics, on the other hand, we need to restore beneficial bacteria in our bodies to-help digestion and promote health balance.

The beneficial bacteria in the human body ideally, about 85 in what we call unbeneficial, or those who may become harmful. These beneficial bacteria help in the absorption of vitamins and minerals during digestion, and thus is an essential part of our natural digestive health. When weighing harmful bacteria, and they take the necessary beneficial bacteria and expel space.

We mentioned antibiotics before because when we take antibiotics for infections of the side effects is that antibiotics often kill beneficial bacteria in the intestines we have. When this happens to displace harmful bacteria beneficial bacteria. This leads to digestive problems.

Probiotics are a way to restore the bacterial balance in the digestive tract.

So how to keep beneficial bacteria probiotics? They do this to flush out other bacteria, bad bacteria that cause intestinal distress. We found good probiotics in foods such as yogurt and other dairy products, used as a preservative. In general, probiotics are a natural way to maintain a healthy balance micro-floral intestine.

Several studies indicate that people are overweight have different intestinal bacteria than thin people. These bacteria cause inflammation of a low grade in the body that makes you gain weight and makes it difficult to lose weight. A family of bacteria called Firmicutes especially helps your body to extract calories from complex sugars and deposit those calories into fat.

Author's Recommendation

To obtain a healthy lifestyle, we highly recommend 65FruitieFibre® Probiotics to include in your daily diet to help weight loss and prevent constipation effectively which lead to colon cancer, visit www.65FruitieFibre.sg

DISCOVER PROVEN STUDY: TAKING PRE AND PROBIOTICS DURING PREGNANCY MAY PREVENT OBESITY AND ASSIST WEIGHT LOSS AFTER BIRTH

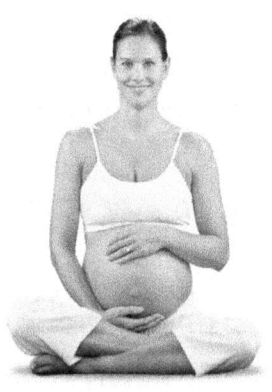 Most women gain a lot of weight during their pregnancy because of their limited knowledge of nutrition.

Most of them are already weighing more than what they should before they even conceive, and that becomes a strenuous problem after their baby birth when they desire to lose their fats.

A recent study took place at the **University of Turku in Finland** by **Kirsi Laitinen** (nutritionist) proved that taking probiotics during an early stage of pregnancy will prevent Obesity and assist weight loss after birth. To study this Kirsi gathered 256 pregnant women and divided them into a group of 3 during their first trimester. All of them were weighed before the start of the study.

The first group was given probiotics along with dietary counseling in which doctors gave the recommendation for beneficial weight gain.

The second group was given dietary counsel too but they received a placebo instead of probiotics. And finally, the third group acted as a control **(Dummy)** and were not given and dietary counseling or supplements.

All the groups continued taking the **probiotics**, **placebo**, and no supplements respectively. At the end of a period of about 12 months when mothers stopped breastfeeding their babies, they were weighed again. Their waist circumference and skin fold thickness were then measured.

Abdominal obesity or **central obesity** is also known as body mass index of 30 or more and weight circumference over 80 centimeters. It was found in 25 percent women who were given probiotics and a regular dietary counsel.

The group which was given dietary counsel alone received a central obesity of 43 percent and those who didn't receive any supplements or **counseling** got a 40 percent of body mass index.

Fat percentage in average was taken out to be **28 percent** in the group taking probiotics, 43 percent who took dietary counseling and **29 percent** in the third group.

Fat belly with abdominal obesity in very unhealthy for mothers' health and the women who got probiotics got the lowest of central obesity even after one year after their childbirth.

The results confirmed the supportive behavior of probiotics in **reducing belly fat** and overall weight loss after birth.

As **Kirsi Laitinen** said:

"The results of our study, the first to demonstrate the impact of probiotics-supplemented dietary counseling on adiposity, were encouraging. The women who got the probiotics fared best.one year after childbirth, they had the lowest levels of central obesity as well as the lowest body fat percentage. There is growing evidence that this approach might open a new angle of the fight against obesity, either through prevention or treatment".

HOW TAKING PROBIOTICS HELP YOUR CHILD:

➢ Protect babies from developing eczema in childhood.

➢ Protect babies from developing eczema in childhood.

➢ Helps to prevent numerous aller-gies during childhood.

➢ Makes your child immune system stronger.

➢ Optimizes the baby's weight later in their life.

➢ Reduces the risk of premature la-bor.

Taking PROBIOTICS can help Mamma in several other ways:

Advantages of Probiotics are not limited, this is versatile and has a waste area of benefits. Probiotics help pregnant women in following ways:

➢ Helps fighting cold and flu.

➢ Prevents constipation.

➢ Optimize pre-eclampsia.

➢ Prevents urinary tract infection.

➢ Prevents yeast infection.

NATURAL FOOD SOURCES OF PRE-BIOTICS:

Following foods have the rich amount of Probiotics in them, in simple words we can say that these foods are worthy eating.

- ➢ Yoghurt.

- ➢ Kefir.

- ➢ Sauerkraut.

- ➢ Pickles.

- ➢ Kimchi.

- ➢ Kombucha tea.

- ➢ Tempeh.

Claim your full bundle eBook (PDF, AZW and Kindle version) at:
http://ebook.65fruitiefibre.sg/bundle

DISCOVER THE FAT AND SUGAR-FREE FOODS TO INCLUDE IN OUR DAILY DIET WHICH HELP IN WEIGHT LOSS

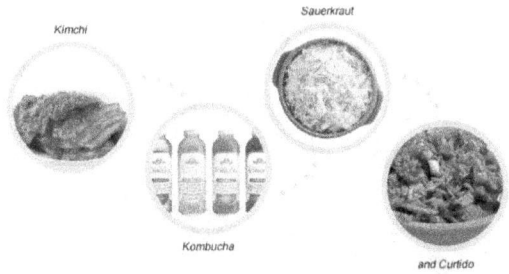

People often miss concept the idea of healthy and **unhealthy fats**, which make them restrict of even good FATS. You must intake the recommended volume of polyunsaturated and monounsaturated while eliminating the use of **saturated fats** and Trans fats, you will find a list below which contains food that is totally fat-free and you must add to your diet to have proper **nutrition** you need with zero fat.

1. Bean:

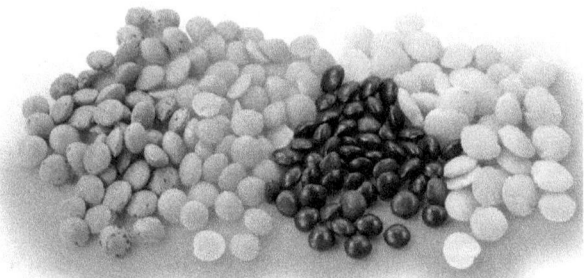

Beans are the main source of high protein and fiber which makes you shed a good amount of calories when you are looking for a diet plan.

A research was carried out in Australia where 42 volunteers were asked to continue their daily diet along with an additional three and a half ounce of chickpeas daily for 12 weeks and then return to their original diet. And the research showed amazing results which proved beans for being essential in weight loss.

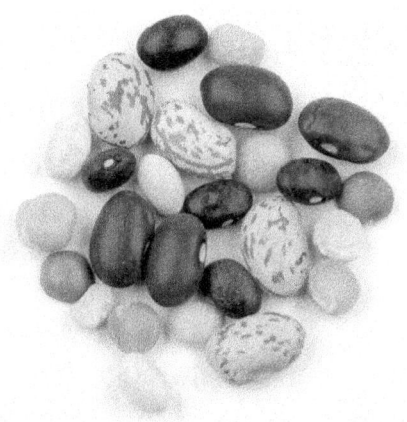

Moreover, a study from the university of Manitoba shows that having beans in your diet boost one's calorie and fat burning to 50 percent!

2. Brown Rice:

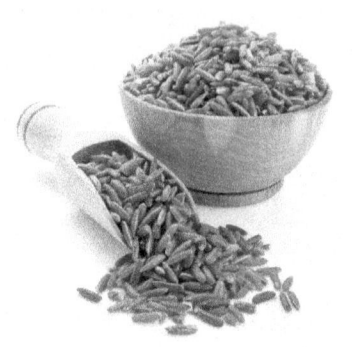

Brown rice aide in weight loss and in controlling obesity. Having high protein and fiber.

A half cup of brown rice contains **110 calories**. Although it's not very helpful in weight loss, but as a substitute for white rice, it's much beneficial. A study has published in Journal of **Nutritional Science** and Vitamin ology in 2014 showed that women who switched to brown rice from white rice improved their blood pressure.

3. Lentils:

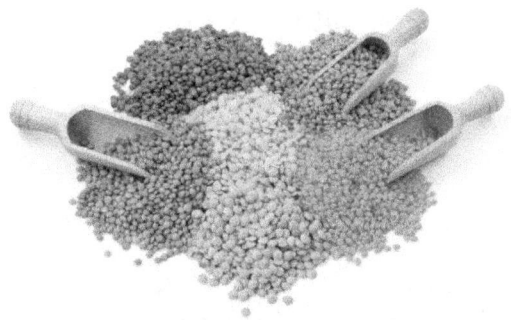

Lentils are the main source of complex carbohydrates that **boosts metabolism** making your fats burn. The high content of fiber in it reduces the cholesterol level. A cup of lentils was tested for its nutrition value and it came up that a cup of it contains 40 grams of **carbo-hydrates**, 18 grams of protein and only 1 gram of fat. They are an excellent substitute for the meal because of their higher content of protein and very **low level of fats**.

Not only will it help you reduce weight but also helps in a good heart health.

4. Green Tea

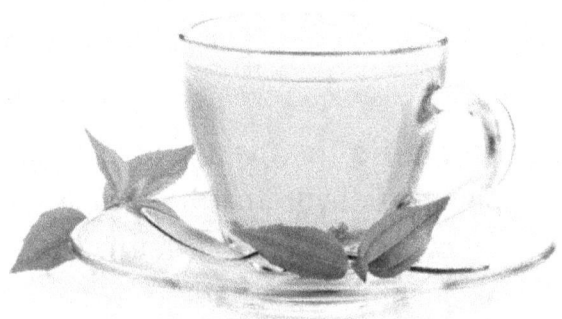

Green tea is also a basic reservoir of complex carbohydrates increase your metabolic rate making it **burn fat**. High fiber which reduces the level of cholesterol in the blood. The cup of green tea for its nutritional value test and reached the cup contains 40 grams of carbohydrates, 18 g protein. They are an excellent alternative to food because of the high content of protein.

Not only will it help you reduce weight but also helps in a good heart health. Green tea is said to be the **healthiest drink** in the world, because of its possession of a high amount of antioxidants and many other health benefits.

In the process of making green tea, bioactive substances in its leaves dissolve to make a final drink. These active compounds boost up the fat burning hormones. It contains little amount of caffeine too. And **caffeine** is also considered aiding weight loss. There are much more benefits of green tea.it contains powerful antioxidants like flavonoids and catechins which reduce the **formation** of free radicals that destroy cells and **molecules** within the body. The minerals in it are important for health.

The stimulant in green tea, "**caffeine**" not only keeps you awake but it will make you look smarter. **Caffeine** makes you feel good, happier, timely reaction and a good memory.

We keep on hearing from the nutritionists that green tea makes you lose weight and increase metabolic rate making you feel more active.

Good metabolism converts fats to energy. Moreover, antioxidants found in green tea will reduce the risk of several types of cancer like breast, prostate and colorectal cancer. Other than this, different research suggested that green tea has different biological benefits too. In a test, green tea was found to kill bacteria and viruses. It kills bacteria in the mouth that causes plaque.

Most **importantly** green tea reduces the chances of type 2 diabetes by reducing blood sugar level and increasing insulin sensitivity.

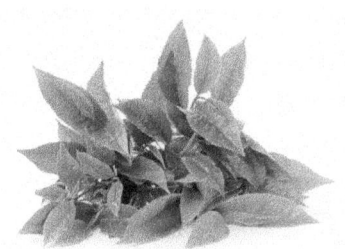

According to 18 types of research, people who consumed green tea had 20 percent fewer chances of being diabetic. Green tea helps you lose weight fast and effectively, especially from the area around the **abdomen**. It prevents from **cardiovascular diseases** like strokes and heart attacks.

Lastly, it's proved that taking green tea will make you live a longer and healthier life as a risk of being obese, diabetic and **cardiovascular** diseases are low.

5. Apples:

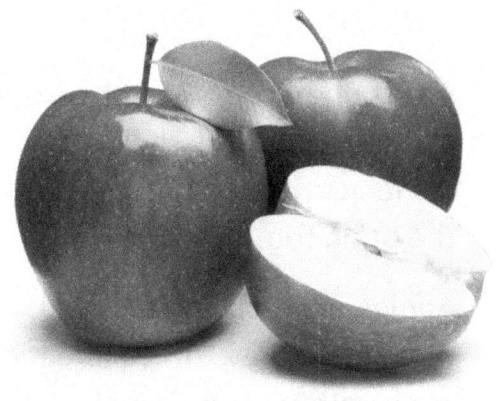

"An Apple a Day Keeps the Doctor Away"

Apple, a 15 in one benefit fruit.

Are you depress of your yellow teeth? That must make you embarrass too. In this case, apple is going to act as your best toothbrush, not only will it make your teeth shine and white but also as strong as an iron rod.

A test on mice showed that drinking apple juice will help one fight Alzheimer and reduce the aging of the brain too.

Apples are rich in flavonoids which reduce the risk of pancreatic cancer.a research in Cornell University proved several compounds in apple peel that fight off cancer cells.

Apples will also decrease the risk of diabetes because of its fibrous nature that lowers the blood sugar. Women who consumed an apple a day were less likely to develop type 2 diabetes. This fiber not only reduces sugar level but also cholesterol level.

By preventing cholesterol and weight, apple helps reduce the formation of gallstones.

Apple will make you beat diarrhea and constipation. Constant constipation leads to irritable bowel, and apple will make it all perfect.

Most of the diseases are caused by being overweight, including heart attack, strokes, and diabetes. To prevent this, doctors recommend taking fiber in the large amount, thus, "**An apple a day keeps the doctor away**". You must have heard this since your childhood. Well, it might not only keep the doctor away but also make you happy on the weighing scale too.

We keep on taking toxins in our daily life by taking normal food and drink. Doctors recommend fruits like apple to detoxify the liver and increase the immune system.

- Apple contains a large amount of fiber when taken it makes you feel full in a stomach and relieve your hunger without gaining a single pound. The fiber that is a non-digestible food source keeps your gut healthy.

- It's recommended to eat in morning.

Author's Recommendation

To obtain a healthy lifestyle, we highly recommend 65FruitieFibre® Probiotics to include in your daily diet to help weight loss and prevent constipation effectively which lead to colon cancer, visit www.65FruitieFibre.sg

Chapter 12

DISCOVER THE SUGAR-FREE FOODS TO INCLUDE IN OUR DAILY LIFE TO PREVENT DIABETES

Diabetes is now becoming a **global epidemic**.

One must be careful in their diet before you get caught by this deadly disease. Nature has provided us with lots of food that helps us in being healthy, getting the nutrition required without consuming large amounts of sugar. Some of the foods that are proved to aid **diabetes prevention** are listed below:

1. Avocado

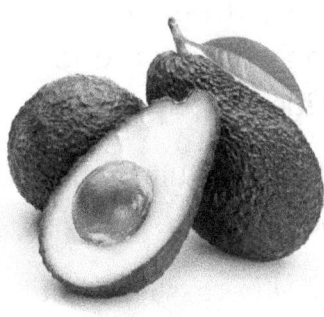

This heavenly fruit is new to the market, but it has made its name in every field of health. By its physical structure, it looks like a pear but its soft taste makes it easier to consume in any way. It can be found in any color from green to black and can weigh from almost 8 ounces to 3 pounds in general.

Avocado contains more than 20 different minerals and vitamins and the most abundantly found in it are Vitamin K, folate, vitamin C, potassium, vitamin B5/B6 and vitamin E.

Magnesium, manganese, iron, copper, zinc and phosphorus are found in lesser quantities.

Avocado is a low-fat fruit with zero cholesterol and sodium.

Potassium is very necessary to build energy in cells, but it's not found commonly in our diets. Avocado is rich in potassium and it contains more potassium than bananas. Potassium regulates blood pressure.

Avocado is a fatty fruit! Now you must be surprised how can it regulate cholesterol and sugar level if it's high in fats. Calm down, because avocado is made up of monounsaturated fatty acid, the same mineral which is found in olive oil and believed to be safe for cooking. Fiber is also a main component of avocado, helping to regulate constipation, reduce blood sugar and help in weight loss.

A study was held to see the effect of avocado on a person. For these two groups were made and one was advised to eat avocado and the other didn't.

The results showed several interests including:

1. Reduction of total cholesterol level

2. Reduction in blood sugar up to 20 percent

3. Increase HDL (good cholesterol) up to 11 percent.

Eating avocado makes you stronger and generate good eyesight.

- AVOCADO is one of the healthiest fruit you will find in nature. Especially if its diabetes we are talking about.

- This beneficial fruit is a high source of monounsaturated fats, vitamin C, potassium and vitamin E.

- So how all these nutrients do are necessary for the control of diabetes?

Monounsaturated fats are considered to be the healthiest fats. They lower the cholesterol level of patients, as they are tolerant to developing heart disease more quickly than a normal healthy person.

- Vitamin C helps a diabetic person in several ways including the improvement of his immune system. It also reduces the chances of heart diseases by its inherent quality of anti-oxidation.

- It helps in the healing of wound too.

2. Broccoli

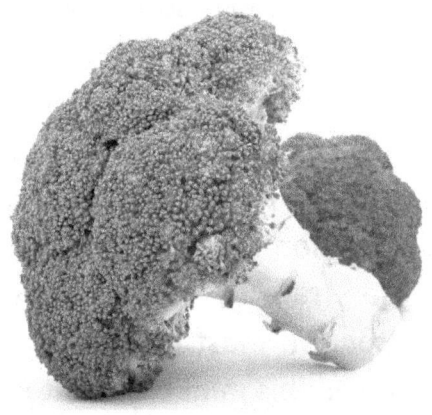

These mini trees have many possible health benefits. Looking in depth of broccoli, many studies have shown that it helps to fight cancer, diabetes and obesity as well. The bitter taste of broccoli is due to sulforaphane in it which is the main cancer-fighting component. Regular intake of broccoli the risk of colon, breast and cervical cancer.

Most people suffer weak bones and complain that they take regular milk but still have brittle bones. Why is that so? Because vitamin K is necessary for the absorption of milk and sadly it's very rare to find in natural food. But you must not be disappointed as this mini tree contains a lot of vitamin K enriched in it.

Which will help your bones stronger?

Now when talking about vitamin C, what's the first thing that comes to your mind? Yes, citrus fruits? You might be astounded to hear that broccoli is a vital source of Vitamin C that makes your skin look fresh and young.

Broccoli is also a source of fiber that will prevent constipation and inflammation. It will remove excess toxins from the bile and stool.

- This vegetable is very credible for combating diabetes due to the high amount of sulforaphane embedded in it.

- It's always recommended to eat a vegetable raw, and same is the case for the intake of broccoli.

- Broccoli is considered one of the favorite vegetables for the prevention of diabetes because of its nutritional qualities

Apart from sulforaphane which helps to reduce the damage to blood vessels by the high amount of sugar in the blood, it is also rich in fiber, vitamins, and minerals.

3. Beans

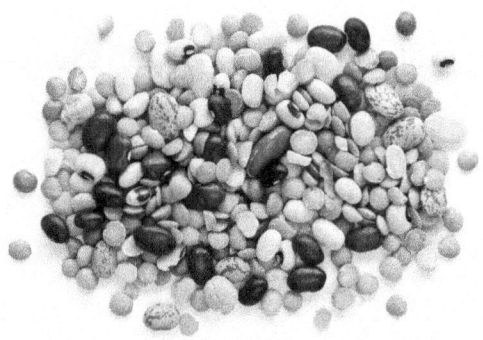

Beans are not considered good by people because of the gas they produce. But researchers say that the more you eat beans the less they'll create gas in you and keep your tummy healthy. To name a few of the beans we have navy beans, kidney beans and black beans. But why are beans so essential? This might not be in our knowledge till now but beans are holding in them a number of benefits.

Talking about few of them, beans are the main source of fiber. Fiber makes the tummy feel full making you eat lesser than usual. Women must intake 25 gram of fiber a day recommends the doctor, but it's true that many of them fall short of it. So taking beans will easily fulfill the daily demand of fiber. Most surprisingly, beans have fiber in their skin as well as the flesh. So when you are using bean you are in taking a good amount of fiber.

Beans consist of soluble and insoluble fiber. Soluble fiber makes the tummy feel full and making you eat lesser while the insoluble fiber prevents constipation.

But while you have beans remember to take a lot of water so that all fiber can be removed from the gut.

Apart from its fibrous nature, beans are pointed as eatables with lowest glycemic index helping to regulate sugar level in blood.

So how they help keep sugar aside? As the beans would digest slowly they'll keep the blood sugar in constant level.

The LDL cholesterol (bad cholesterol) often stick to the walls of blood vessels, so when beans are injected the fibrous compound binds with the cholesterol helping it not to dissolve in blood. Those who intake ¾ cup of lentils a day they have 5 percent of chances to develop cardiovascular diseases.

It's also good for your heart when one percent of cholesterol decreases, two percent of the risk of heart attack decreases.

Beans contain potassium and mineral which are essential elements for the wealth of your heart. Potassium neutralize excess sodium in the body making the blood pressure lower naturally.

Let's come to another beneficial component of beans that is it's highly rich in protein. Protein and fiber together delay stomach emptiness and delays your demand of hunger. Beans are low fat in nature, which makes it easier for you to lose weight.

Are you dealing with iron deficiency? Yes, you might be, one in every 5 people around the globe is dealing with low HB level. Now how does that link to beans? The very cheap vegetables in the market. Surprised? Beans are rich in iron and if any of you women is dealing with low HB start a diet containing beans.

But make sure you take Vitamin C along with beans as its non-home iron and can't be absorbed by itself. Vitamin C will together help to get incorporate in blood. It will make the absorption 6 times more than it will naturally. Now you must not need to take vitamin C supplements, instead try your diet with beans along with tomato or broccoli, which are rich in vitamin C.

4. Berries:

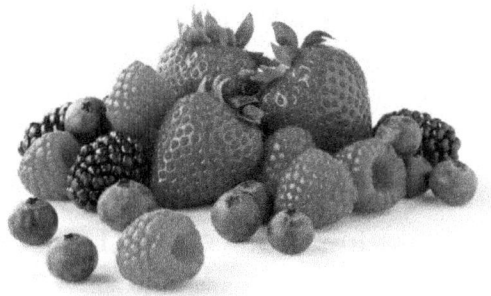

Extremely high in antioxidants, every day new examinations are suggesting numerous health benefits of berries. Let's take a look at it discussing their benefits in regards to different species of berries.

The deep Blueberries are a hub of antioxidants with possessing a large number of phytonutrients called anthocyanidins. The anthocyanidins help to neutralize the radical damage on the cell. A recent study at Tufts University analyzed 50 fruits and vegetables for their antioxidant behavior and this blueberry was ranked number one in it. Blueberries help to fight any disease related to redness of cells including heart diseases.

A study in American Institute of cancer research announced that the antioxidant power of blueberry can be helpful for a body to delay the risk of cancer.

Goji berries are often linked with sexual vitality, happiness, and physical strength. They are found in Nepal and are considered a good fruit when one is suffering contamination of liver. This dark red fruit has responded well for a cancer patient. Its components include amino acid, minerals, vitamin B and germanium.

5. Carrots:

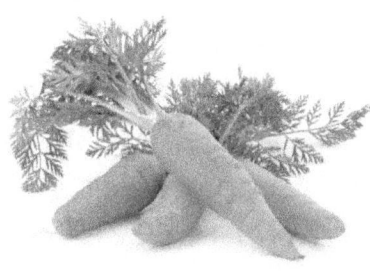

Carrots! Yes, it might seem to you an ordinary vegetable, mostly used for salads or eating raw and always seen in red or orange color. Let us first give you the most surprising fact about carrots. These carrots are not only occurring as red or orange, around the world in different regions you can find them in white, yellow, red, or even purple colored. Did you know? Carrots can be farmed as small as two inches or as long as three whole feet! Isn't that amazing? Apart from this astounding physical occurrences carrots hold an amazing amount of treasure in them. And the one recently discovered, after a 10-year study in Netherlands is that eating carrots can reduce the risk of cardiovascular diseases. Participants of this study who took carrots were considered to have less risk of cardiovascular diseases.

Most of us around are aware of the beneficiary worth of the carrot being a hub of antioxidants, which supports burn fats. Not particularly this, a contemporary study showed the presence of falcarinol in it. Components that prevent colon cancer!

This crunchy root vegetable will help you feel full of tummy, without raising your blood glucose level due to its low glycemic index of 97 whereas regular sugar is considered to have 100.

The beneficial nutrients absorbed in carrots will provide you with vitamin A, vitamin K. vitamin C, and potassium, and manganese, complex vitamin B, with folate, phosphorus, and vitamin E.

Claim your full bundle eBook (PDF, AZW and Kindle version) at:
http://ebook.65fruitiefibre.sg/bundle

Chapter 13

WANT TO KNOW THE SECRET TO LOOKING SLIM AND BEAUTIFUL? ONE MUST READ THIS

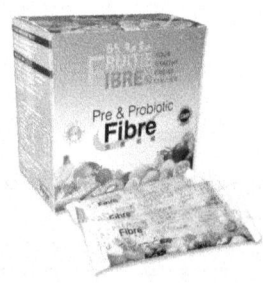

It's sure that this book must have helped you in escalating the knowledge towards pre and probiotics and their benefits in numerous ways including their assistance towards diabetes control and weight loss.

We served you by recommending best weight loss tips and diet plan, best diabetes control diet, and tips too.

This book primarily summarized how probiotics can help reduce pregnancy weight gain. You might have felt doubting yourself that can these microorganisms actually be so effective for us, hence this theory was proved by the premium researches done around the world.

*So what are you waiting
for, get your desired body
back by using
65FruitieFibre®
Probiotics.*

Its ingredients include:

- ✓ **Psyllium husk**
- ✓ **Fruits and vegetable powder**
- ✓ **Chlorophyll**
- ✓ **Prebiotics**
- ✓ **Guar gum**
- ✓ **Lactose**

- ✓ **Probiotics (Bifidobacterium)**
- ✓ **Crystalline fructose**
- ✓ **Passion fruit flavor**
- ✓ **Citric acid**

65FruitieFibre® Probiotics is approved by the authority of Singapore

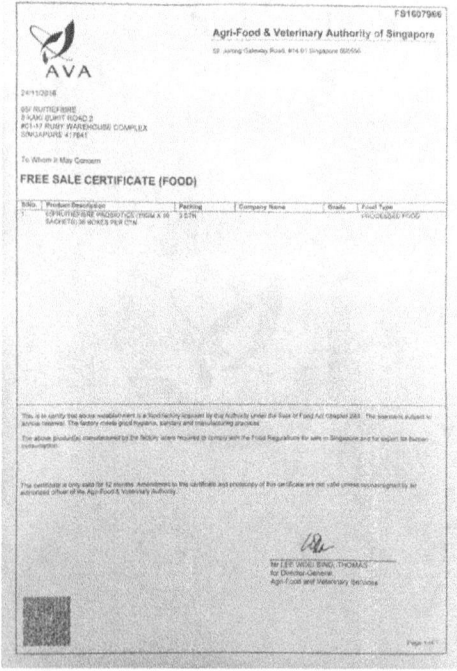

Conclusion

65FruitieFibre® Probiotics is a versatile and dynamic product. Moreover, 65FruitieFibre® Probiotics is the most effective and finest product you can find in the market. With the efforts of our scientists and great research, we are blessed to offer this product to our honorable and respected clients. Keeping all the proportion of constituents in eye, this 65FruitieFibre® Probiotics is utterly beneficial for users. Having no side effects, this product is favorable in all aspects of healthy life. We hope and we believe, you will get your desired results by using our product.

About The Author, 65FruitieFibre® Team:

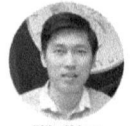 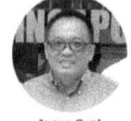 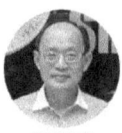 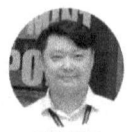

Billy Chiam   Jason Seah   Andy Low   Wilson Tan

65FruitieFibre® is a privately owned Singapore company specializing in the distribution and exporting of natural health products. It is a homegrown brand from Singapore. 65FruitieFibre® Pre and Probiotics Fiber has proven to be safe and reliable for everyday consumption and approved by AVA, Authority of Singapore.

Our Values:

Your health comes first. The reason why we make probiotics supplements in sachets is because we strongly believe this is the most effective way to have your probiotics.

Many probiotics yogurt drinks have extremely high doses of sugar which can be damaging to our health. Light versions of these drinks often contain artificial sweeteners such as aspartame and the chemical containing toxic effects which are harmful to the human body.

65FruitieFibre® Probiotics products are rich in nutrient and vitamins and free from artificial sweeteners and nasty additives. Everyone deserves a good health. Money can't buy good health no matter how much money we have. 65FruitieFibre® Probiotics proven to help different people to achieve a healthy lifestyle. If you are looking for pre and probiotics support for bowel calm, detoxification or to maintain a flat stomach, we offer a condition-specific combination of probiotics strains.

Our Motto:

If we are healthy, the world belongs to us. 65FruitieFibre® Probiotics are made from natural ingredients with the most advanced biotechnological techniques. They are natural, simple to consume, effective, efficient, safe and free from adverse side effects.

People of all ages can safely consume 65FruitieFibre® Probiotics, including pregnant women and children, to consume these products for the enhancement of their health and vitality in the shortest possible time.

If We Are Healthy, the World Belong To us.

We are reachable anytime for our respected clients. Don't hesitate to contact us.

Phone: Billy Chiam: (65) 97818351 and Jason Seah (65) 90661328

Visit Our Website:

http://www.65fruitiefibre.sg

For Facebook users:

https://www.facebook.com/65fruitiefibre/